THE NEW
HIATUS H

A naturopathic practitioner provides advice on the
causes of this distressing ailment and its successful
alleviation using a programme of self-help, natural,
drug-free treatments.

By the same author
DIETS TO HELP COLITIS

THE <u>NEW</u> SELF HELP SERIES

HIATUS HERNIA

Avoid or alleviate this common complaint by
making the change to a healthier lifestyle

by
Joan Lay N.D., M.B.N.O.A.

THORSONS PUBLISHERS LIMITED
Wellingborough, Northamptonshire

First published 1982
This revised, enlarged and reset edition, 1986

British Library Cataloguing in Publication Data

Lay, Joan
  Hiatus hernia: avoid or alleviate this common
  complaint by making the change to a healthier
  lifestyle.—Rev., enl. and reset ed.
  1. Naturopathy   2. Hiatal hernia
  I. Title   II. Lay, Joan. Self-help for hiatus hernia
  617.559065   RZ440

  ISBN 0-7225-1222-8

Printed and bound in Great Britain

Contents

INTRODUCTION:

What is Hiatus Hernia?

The medical definition of hiatus hernia is: 'displacement of a portion of the stomach through the opening in the diaphragm through which the oesophagus passes from the chest to the abdominal cavity.' To put it another way: a part of the upper wall of the stomach protrudes through the diaphragm at the point where the gullet passes from the chest area to the abdominal area.

The diaphragm is a large, dome-shaped muscle, dividing the chest from the abdominal cavity. It is the muscle concerned with breathing, and it is assisted by the intercostal muscles (those between the ribs) during exertion. It has special openings in it to allow for the passage of important blood vessels (the aorta and the vena cava) and for the food channel (the oesophagus). It is the oesophageal opening (hiatus) that concerns us here, because this is the point where the hernia occurs.

Such hernias become increasingly common after middle age, and it is estimated that about half the population of over sixty years of age suffers from them, although often without any symptoms. A barium X-ray is required for exact diagnosis, but a qualified diagnosis can be arrived at through the recognition of various

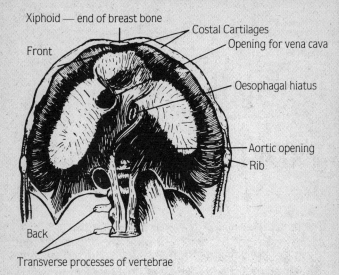

Xiphoid — end of breast bone
Costal Cartilages
Opening for vena cava
Front
Oesophagal hiatus
Aortic opening
Rib
Back
Transverse processes of vertebrae

Figure 1: The diaphragm, seen from below

symptoms. Hiatus hernia is characterized by pain in several areas. The commonest are behind the sternum (breast bone) at nipple level; and lower, behind the xiphoid process, at the end of the breast bone. Other areas of pain can be located on the left chest and may be mistaken for angina; at the base of the throat, or the right lower-ribs; and, more rarely, through the back behind the right shoulder blade.

Hiccups are sometimes symptomatic due to irritation of the phrenic nerve when the hernia is a large one. Pain increases on stooping with effort, and on lying down. 'Heartburn' is the usual description of the pain, and this is always worse after a meal. There is usually a feeling of fullness and bloatedness, and a considerable amount of flatulence is experienced. Intermittent nausea is sometimes complained of, and projectile vomiting can occur in severe cases.

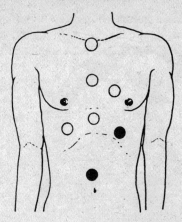

Figure 2: Different sites of pain

As you will learn from the following pages, the holistic approach to healing certainly requires time and application, if not dedication. However, the means of treatment are simple and they are safe.

Repressive treatment that is aimed mainly at relieving symptoms only prolongs the condition. In this case the patient may feel more comfortable, but nothing is being done to treat the cause, and most drug treatment produces side-effects of some sort. In addition, the body has to deal with the drugs whilst in a depleted or 'ill' state. This, in turn, increases the drain on vitality and further weakens the organism.

On the other hand, with natural treatment, after a short time patients are aware of a feeling of well-being and increased energy, even though there is still a lot to do, and some symptoms may persist. There is a feeling of 'rightness' about the regime which will give you an encouragement to persevere. Many patients have said that they had no idea how well they could feel, until they had tried natural healing.

The holistic approach is a way of life and not just aimed at curing conditions. By following this sensible plan, and then adopting it, with some adaptations, for the future, much ill health will be prevented. It is certainly my sincere hope that you will be encouraged to change your way of life, not just for the treatment of your hiatus hernia but to improve your standard of health over all.

1.

The Causes of Hiatus Hernia

In naturopathic circles there is no doubt that the mechanical defect associated with hiatus hernia is caused by such factors of twentieth-century western civilization as: sedentary occupations, overweight, smoking and shallow breathing, impoverished diet, tight clothing and mental and emotional tension.

Sedentary Occupations

Without sensible — that is, regular — exercise, the system is predisposed to various types of ailments because cell activity is diminished. This means that elimination of waste matter is slowed and incomplete. Assimilation of nutrients is also retarded and so metabolism is at a lower level. This results in toxic matter accumulating in the body, and in functional quality being reduced.

It is *not* a good idea to offset a sedentary job by violent exertion at weekends. Too much stress and strain is then thrust upon a body which is unprepared and unfit for strenuous activity. Steady, progressive training is the best plan, but if this is not possible then gentler exercise, such as non-competitive walking or swimming should be included in the weekly routine. Too much reliance on the car and lack of physical activity at work is responsible for many mechanical difficulties in the body, including spinal problems, varicose veins, constipation and so on, although these are also associated with an impoverished dietetic background.

Overweight

This is due to overeating; whether it be nibbling between meals, or eating too much at meal times, or a combination of both. Large meals are the greater danger in the condition we are discussing, because they increase the mechanical pressure on the diaphragm from the greatly distended stomach. However, overweight is always debilitating and taxing on the body, and it leads to dimimished cell activity, reduced metabolism and a general 'below par' feeling. The adipose (fatty) tissue also mechanically compresses the diaphragm and abdominal organs from without, inhibiting movement and proper organic function, often resulting in constipation which intensifies the toxic state.

Smoking and Shallow Breathing

Smoking is a menace in any condition. It is by now an accepted fact that lung cancer is caused by smoking. But even aside from this the *entire* level of health is lowered by the impoverished air circulating in the lungs and therefore in the bloodstream which, as a result, is unable to take oxygen to the tissues, or to absorb all the carbon dioxide from them. The absorption of vitamin B is inhibited and so the nervous system is made more vulnerable. This creates a vicious circle since smoking is erroneously thought to 'steady' the nerves. When lack of exercise coincides with the intake of stodgy, over-refined and rich foods, it can be seen how the interconnected systems are put at considerable risk, and prevented from producing anything approaching well-being and wholeness.

Shallow breathing may be a result of smoking, or it may be caused by tight clothing, or by tension through daily pressures and anxiety. Shallow breathing occurs when the diaphragm is held tightly and only the upper chest moves during inhalation and exhalation. Therefore, due to lack of use, or little use, the muscle tone is diminished and so renders the diaphragm more liable to herniation. Added to this, shallow breathing inadequately aerates the lungs, and this results in less toxic elimination and less absorption of oxygen. Thorough interchange of gases in the lungs is essential to good health.

It can easily be understood, then, that smoking and shallow breathing predispose the 'victim' to many disorders: respiratory, digestive, circulatory and nervous.

Impoverished Diet
There are so many unwholesome ingredients in products which come under the heading of 'food' today: for instance, the refined white flour contained in so many cakes, biscuits and breads; preservatives in meat, including sausages and delicatessen salamis; chemicals, improvers and flavourings added to ice-cream and squashes — not to mention refined sugar and syrups and an excess of salt in many packeted and easy-cook products such as instant mashed potato, custard powders and so on.

All these things should be avoided, since eating much devitalized and refined foods results in far less oxygen being introduced into the body than is required. Fewer mineral salts and vitamins are made available to balance and activate proper nutrition and, in addition, there is too little fibre present to stimulate the peristaltic action of the colon and keep it healthy. As a result, all body tissues function at less than their full potential — indeed, at less than their average potential. Muscle tone is weakened, and the muscles become less resilient, and connective and fibrous tissue suffers through poor nourishment, and is consequently more prone to atrophy and damage. Also the mucous membranes become thinned and more easily irritated.

Drinks, too, can be harmful. Tea and coffee both irritate the nervous system and the digestive tract, and leave acid wastes that slow down elimination. Squashes, coffee, and alcohol all affect the mucous lining of the stomach. When these drinks are taken with meals, or immediately afterwards, the weight of the stomach content is increased, stretching the stomach wall. This unwise mixture also encourages fermentation and produces gas; thus the distension of the stomach is increased, causing pressure against the diaphragm and the oesophageal opening, and greatly increasing the risk of herniation.

'We are what we eat', so it is up to every individual to eat a fully balanced diet which provides the body with all the necessary raw materials for its proper function. In this way health is maintained and disease prevented. A healthy regime should consist of *at least* fifty per cent fruit and vegetables, and at least half of that amount should be uncooked. The other food categories — carbohydrates, proteins and fats — should make up the other fifty per cent. When we really do eat and drink wisely, the functional standard of every system in the body improves. As a result we think more clearly and act with greater precision and awareness.

In many cases of hiatus hernia it has been found that air-swallowing is a factor which exacerbates the condition by distending the stomach. This usually occurs when air is gulped in with food. One way of avoiding this is to remember to breathe *out* each time food is put into the mouth.

Tight Clothing

Restriction of movement around the waist causes compression. This reacts on the digestive, nervous and circulatory systems, but particularly on the diaphragm and respiratory system. Movement is restricted, and the body functions are undermined. Some women, for example, choose to wear a bra and girdle which overlap at the waist to control a 'spare tyre'. Though this may achieve its objective, such clothing is really detrimental to health, and is a strong predisposing factor in the condition of hiatus hernia.

Mental and Emotional Tension

All emotional and mental tensions and upsets react on the vagus nerve and sympathetic nervous system. The most easily recognized area affected is the solar plexus — where the feeling of 'butterflies' occurs when we are anxious. In such instances the solar plexus tightens up and the feeling experienced is like a hard lump. Most of us know the horrible sick feeling experienced when we pass an accident on the road. Jealousy, anger, resentment and self-pity all react on this finely tuned 'relay station' whose function is to get adrenalin flowing and to increase the heartbeat and rate of blood-flow. Further metabolic changes include faster breathing to correspond with an increased pulse rate, and the retardation of the digestive functions and the repair and growth processes. When chronic anxiety occurs all this takes place, though less noticeably, diminishing function and inhibiting diaphragmatic movement, which is so essential to good health and the prevention of hiatus hernia.

2.

Relaxation

What can be done to treat this distressing ailment? It is obviously necessary to rehabilitate the whole body; a momentous task indeed but, taken slowly, step by step, with a positive persistence, the new regime will not be too difficult and, as the body systems are relieved, you will experience the encouragement to persevere. Before beginning the actual treatment, it is a wise idea to raise the head end of the bed, either by using bricks on which to stand the legs of the bed, or by wedging the mattress higher, using a very firm bolster, a piece of wood or wedge-shaped foam rubber. (More pillows can also be used.) This will help prevent the regurgitation of food during the night and relieve flatulence and heartburn.

First, it is important to learn to breathe properly; that is, using the diaphragm. By doing this you will begin to relax. Diaphragmatic breathing is really quite easy, and the following routine is to be recommended.

Lie down with both knees bent and feet close to buttocks; relax your body, put both hands lightly on the abdomen (*note:* this is not shown in the diagram, to avoid obscuring the abdominal movements) and concentrate the attention on this area. Now breathe in, gently pushing the abdomen up under the hands at the same time, until no more air can be inhaled. Then relax, breathing out through the mouth with an audible sighing sound and allowing the abdominal wall to sink back (see diagram). The shoulders and chest should remain at rest throughout.

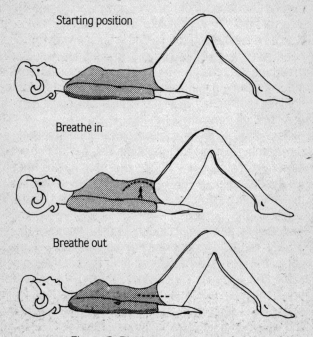

Starting position

Breathe in

Breathe out

Figure 3: Diaphragmatic breathing

At first, there might be a desire to 'suck in' the abdomen and expand the chest, because this is what is understood by 'deep breathing', and some methods of teaching emphasize chest expansion as the most important part of respiration. It certainly does play a part, but the use of the diaphragm increases the capacity of the lungs by utilizing the deeper lung tissue. Rhythmical movement, or athletic training to increase lung capacity, exerts a massaging effect on the abodominal organs, stimulating good function.

A really complete breath begins with the diaphragm and continues with the intercostal muscles which expand the lungs from above, downwards, and from side to side. Try a complete breath once or twice. It would be exhausting to breathe in such a way for long, but it is very useful in exercising. In everyday conditions, breathing is a reflex action and, unless the diaphragm is influenced in a negative way — by anxiety, tension or holding the tummy in for the sake of appearance, it performs its function well.

Back, then, to the practice. It is best done first thing in the morning and last thing at night. Begin with five or six 'tummy' breaths, increasing by one each day to fifteen. Always be at ease — do not use force. If any strain is felt, then too much effort is being exerted; working hard at it defeats the purpose. Get up slowly afterwards (especially after the morning session), as deep breathing usually causes a slight feeling of giddiness. This is normal, and is due to acceleration of the circulation and passes off after a few seconds. During the day, just occasionally, try to do the same type of breathing while sitting, well supported, in a chair; then, while standing and walking. However, don't worry if it doesn't seem to work. The very action of directing thought to the diaphragm helps to promote its function, and the exercise will get easier each time. This type of breathing will relieve pain, so it should be practised whenever there is an attack.

It is important to be able to relax at any time since, through the learning and application of this skill, it is possible to prevent bodily and mental tensions from building up into proportions that cause actual physical symptoms. To begin then, lie down on a hard surface (though it may be uncomfortable to start with, it is more difficult to cheat yourself and has more teaching value than a soft bed or couch). A sleeping bag laid on the floor is good or, in fine summer weather, a rug on the garden lawn would be splendid — relaxation is impossible in cold conditions.

Part of the art of relaxation is learning to be aware of the body in a positive way. With real awareness comes the ability to recognize stress-tension at once, and the build-up cannot occur if the stress is released in the first instance. To make the contrast between tension and relaxation more vivid to the learner, a series of deliberate actions of tensing and releasing several different muscle and joint groups is practised, beginning with the feet and working up to the head. It is done in harmony with the breathing, in this manner:

1. Breathe in, and bend the feet up to ninety degrees. Hold for a few seconds, noting the tautness in the shin muscles and ankle joints. Breathe out to a sigh and 'let go' — don't try to *do* anything in this half of the movement, simply release the tension caused by bending the feet up. Repeat once.
2. Move your attention up to the knees. Breathe in as you press both knees on to the ground, noting the tautness in the thigh muscles. Breathe out to a sigh and release them. Repeat.
3. Move your attention to the buttocks. Breathe in and contract (squeeze) these muscles together. (Try not to tighten any other area of the body. You may catch yourself clenching hands or jaws to 'assist', but this must be prevented.) Note the tension as before, and then release it while breathing out and sighing. Repeat.

4. Think about your abdominal area (tummy). Draw these muscles back, as if to touch your spine while breathing in (the reverse of diaphragmatic breathing). Hold for a few seconds, noticing the discomfort, and then breathe out and release the muscles. Repeat.

5. The hands are next on the list — clench them both really tightly, increasing the grip as you breathe in — you can really feel the 'blocking' that tension will cause. Breathe out sighing and release the hands. It should give quite a sense of relief if the clenching was strong. Repeat.

6. Bend the elbows hard, hands up to shoulders, breathing in — breathe out and release as before. Repeat.

7. Next, while breathing in, draw the shoulder blades together tightly, note the discomfort, and release it while sighing. Repeat.

8. Now the face muscles — screw up the muscles around the eyes, frown, and clench the jaw, all while breathing in. Then release with a sigh. Repeat.

9. Finish off this preliminary section by adding all the 'tensings' together and stiffen the whole body, then 'fall in a heap', so to speak, while releasing and sighing out. Repeat.

It takes quite an effort to do this, and the relief of letting go is very noticeable. Follow this with three or four slow, deep diaphragmatic breaths, still sighing as you breathe out. Begin to still your mind by deliberately remembering a beautiful place — somewhere special to you — quiet and deserted, and, in imagination, put yourself there. Explore it in your mind's eye and appreciate its beauty deeply; feel yourself as part of this beauty. Ignore your body, and expand into these lovely surroundings. Imagine yourself to be part of the universe (which you are), essential in the scheme of things. Get to the stage where you feel contented, at peace, warm and drowsy and just stay there for a few minutes (or as long as you can). Everyday thoughts will pop into your mind from time to time unbidden; try to let them float through without getting annoyed or pursuing them, and return to your visualized beautiful place. Gradually, the active mind will become calmed, and the interfering thoughts will decrease and eventually cease; though this may take several weeks of practice. When you are ready, leave the lovely place, come back to the present, yawn and stretch and 'wake up'. Get up gradually because resting slows down metabolism and to hurry up might involve a slight shock to the system.

Incidentally, if you are within hearing of a telephone, either bury it in cushions or take it off the hook. As you can understand, the aim of all this is to become completely detached from everyday things for a while, and allow mind and body to rest and recharge. Practised every day, taking ten, then twenty, minutes and working up to half an hour, your conscious mind, and also the subconscious will be trained and, in time, you will realize that you are not getting so uptight about things, that worry doesn't penetrate so deeply and that you are calmer. This regime is tremendously helpful in any condition where anxiety and tension are factors.

3.

DIET

Now we come to the point where preconceived ideas have to be unlearnt and new thoughts adopted; so it is necessary to be willing to adopt a fresh outlook and to try out the new approach with an open mind.

Habits and Addictions
Begin, if you smoke, by giving up or, if you find it easier, cut down by two cigarettes a day, steadily. Although this will prove difficult, keep in mind the fact that the whole body is going to benefit once the withdrawal problems are over. Allow one cup (not mug) of coffee substitute and one cup of tea each day. At other times, have fruit or vegetable juices, herbal teas or beverages such as *Barley Cup* or a dandelion coffee. There is a wide choice, all obtainable at health food shops. At the same time, remember to observe separate eating and drinking times; take fluids half an hour before a meal, or two hours afterwards. This helps the digestive process considerably and reduces the incidence of heartburn. Drinking with meals increases the overall weight in the stomach, slows down the digestive process by diluting the digestive juices and thus increases the risk of

fermentation and gas formation, which distends the stomach and causes pressure and, therefore, discomfort and pain.

All meals should be smaller in quantity than usual, and thorough mastication is essential, both to break up the food into really small particles, and to slow down the rate of intake. A rough estimate would be about thirty-two to forty chews for each mouthful. Please do *not* count every mouthful eaten. Be conscious of chewing more thoroughly and, now and then, count, just to see how near the mark you get. Obviously, it will depend on the type of food eaten, and this introduces another point; on the whole, the diet will consist of more fruit and vegetables than before and less soft, refined, and over-processed things like white bread and sugar, cakes and biscuits, rice puddings and overcooked vegetables. I mentioned at the beginning, and repetition will help to emphasize, that diets in general should consist of at least fifty per cent fruit and vegetables, and fifty per cent, collectively, of protein, carbohydrates and fat.

Raw Juices

In the case of the hiatus hernia, it is very important to introduce raw juices into the diet as soon as possible. However, the digestive tract will probably be hypersensitive at first; therefore, it is suggested that raw, freshly-made carrot juice be sipped half an hour before each meal, even before breakfast. Even without a juice extractor it can still be prepared quite simply, and instructions can be found, together with sample menus and recipes, later in this book. Carrot juice has a very restorative effect, as it is rich in vitamin A and calcium, and is also an alkaline substance, which soothes the stomach. Persevere with this even though, admittedly, carrot juice tastes rather insipid. Note here that all juices, whether fruit or vegetable, should be slightly diluted because they are somewhat concentrated. Always add one tablespoon of water to each 4 fl oz (120 ml) of juice; either tap or bottled water can be used. Variations can be made later, by mixing fresh apple juice with the carrot, and by using beetroot and apple juice together, or beetroot and celery — though these latter really need a proper juicer. The bottled varieties of fruit juice are quite good, but they have had to be pasteurized, so some vitamin and oxygen content is lost. Nevertheless, it is a quick and clean way of obtaining juices.

It is worth mentioning that beetroots, eaten in any quantity, cause coloration of the urine (pink) and faeces (dark red). This is normal, and not a symptom of disease.

General Principles of Healthy Eating

Eat only wholefoods; that is, only those things that have not had their original goodness refined out of them, as is the case with white flour, white rice and so on.

Eat those foods that have not been contaminated with unnecessary flavourings, colourings, 'improvers', preservatives, or heavy salt and sugar additives. The inclusion of food additives such as these has to be stated on packages or tins by law — *so read your labels!*

Tinned meat and fish are usually heavily salted or treated with preservatives, so be careful of these — also highly spiced and preserved delicatessen meats. Many cheeses are high in salt, so check for low-sodium varieties or brands.

Eat generously of fruits and salads, nuts, seeds, grains and pulses and all vegetables. Dried fruits are good but are rather concentrated, so need to be eaten carefully balanced with fresh fruit or mineral water.

Meat, poultry, fish, eggs, cheese — *all* proteins — need to be offset with *plenty* of vegetables to maintain a reasonable acid/alkali balance.

I have already said that any diet should consist of fifty per cent vegetables and fruit, to balance the acidity of the other fifty per cent foodstuffs, namely the carbohydrates, proteins and fats.

The average diet pays far too much attention to protein: 2-4 oz (55-115 g) per day is ample for anyone not involved in hard, physical work. There are plenty of other sources of protein in the vegetables, seeds, grains and pulses.

More attention needs to be paid to *balance* in a diet, so that vitamins, minerals and fibre all play a part. In this way the body will get the optimum amount of the materials needed to function healthily.

Enjoyment of food is also important, and dishes that are attractive-looking stimulate the digestive juices to increase the pleasure in eating the food and aid digestion.

Eating in a relaxed atmosphere, having time to eat slowly, chewing the food properly; all have been mentioned before, but form the basis of good digestion and should be remembered.

Your New Diet

It is a good plan to begin the day well by introducing something beneficial into the body. So instead of the usual cup of tea, which over-stimulates the nervous system, irritates the lining of the stomach, and increases acidity in the blood stream, have a herbal tea. These have a gentler effect and activate the healing resources of the body. Peppermint tea aids digestion, disperses flatulence and tones up the lining of the stomach.

Chamomile soothes the nervous system and is good for colic; so either is excellent first thing in the morning and, taken alternately, you get the benefits of both.

Always allow hot drinks to cool a little before consuming. Extremes of temperature, in both food and drink, should be avoided; and just as food should be eaten slowly, so drinks should be sipped.

Some readers may find it better suited to their particular temperament and the regime of the home to make these changes slowly. Natural processes are slow, and it is far better to make alterations gradually and consistently, than to rush into a situation and then find yourself unable to maintain it. In addition, too many sudden changes can cause a reaction in the body, perhaps temporarily increasing symptoms, which could act as a deterrent to further dieting.

Week One
Use this week as follows:

1. Learn the breathing and relaxation techniques.
2. Drink 4 fl oz (120 ml) of freshly made carrot juice before each meal. Remember, this should be *sipped.*
3. Drink and eat at separate times.
4. If necessary, cut out (or down) smoking.
5. Drink only one cup of tea and one cup of coffee substitute per day.
6. Begin the day with peppermint or chamomile tea.
7. Eat smaller meals, and chew them very well.
8. Raise the bed-head level by four to six inches (10-15 cm) and generally get into the feel of the new regime. Prepare to let the natural forces in the body take over and redress the imbalance that has been going on for so long and, in time, all these eight

factors cannot fail to produce improvement; indeed, any one of them would help a little.

The second week will involve following a stricter plan, aimed at cleansing the body of toxic wastes and stimulating repair processes, at the same time relieving pain and discomfort.

The diet will be very simple at first, using natural wholefoods and few mixtures, as an aid to digestion. Gradually, more foods that are rich in oxygen, vitamins and minerals will be introduced, to promote healing and health. A full diet, based on wholefoods, of course, and preferably vegetarian, will then be suggested at the end of the course. This phase, the last one concerning the hiatus hernia, will be the first phase of a new way of life, with no going back to the old, unhealthy habits. It should be a life of increased vitality, and greater capacity both for work and enjoyment; a life of broader concepts and spiritual awareness; a life of sound health.

Week Two

The basic food for the week is brown rice because it contains silica, a mineral which helps the body to eliminate toxic matter and also helps to initiate healing, especially in digestive problems. Brown rice still retains its natural bran, which is more delicate than wheat bran, and so provides bulk for the system without irritation. Rice is largely a starch food, but it has about eight per cent protein content, as well as traces of calcium and phosphorous and, more importantly, several of the B vitamins — thiamine, niacin and, to a lesser extent, riboflavin. These vitamins are valuable in nourishing the nervous system, as is well known.

The three main meals will be rice-based. The grain is boiled, and it will save a lot of effort if sufficient is cooked to last for two days. Wash half a pound (225g) of rice in a sieve, and drop it into one pint (570ml) of boiling water, to which one teaspoon of sunflower oil has been added. (This helps to keep the grains separate.) Allow to boil slowly, until all the moisture has been absorbed — about twenty to twenty-five minutes. Turn out into a basin or container with a lid, and it is ready; keep in the fridge or a cool place. The amount recommended will be small, deliberately so, but if you are really needing more, a little extra may be added.

Week Two, Day One:

7 a.m. On waking, peppermint or chamomile tea.

8 a.m. 4 fl oz (120 ml) freshly made carrot juice.

8.30 a.m. Breakfast: 3 level tablespoons of boiled rice; 3 tablespoons of stewed apple sweetened with honey (this may be warmed up if preferred).

10.30 a.m. Barley Cup.

12.30 p.m. Carrot juice.

1 p.m. Lunch: 3 tablespoons of rice with 1 tablespoon of finely grated raw carrot and 1 tablespoon of finely chopped parsley. (This provides vitamins A and C, calcium and potassium.) A very little yeast extract or soya sauce can be added.

3 p.m. China tea or herb tea.

5 p.m. Carrot juice.

5.30 p.m. Evening meal: 3 tablespoons of rice with 4 to 6 prunes or apricots that have been soaked overnight, not cooked, and 2 tablespoons of natural yogurt.

7.30 p.m. Barley Cup or herb tea, followed, half an hour before bedtime, by 4 fl oz (120 ml) red grape juice with a generous splash of mineral water. This is a good sedative drink and a digestive as well.

Sleep should be good when following this plan, as there will be no food in the stomach by bedtime; and by having the night drink half an hour before going to bed, that too will be well on its way through the digestive tract. Diaphragmatic breathing will also help to induce sleep.

Week Two, Day Two:
This is a repetition of the first day, though amounts may need to be varied a little. It is important that the lower bowel be kept free; and, as the total amount of bulk being taken in is less than usual, there may be temporary constipation. If this second day passes without any motion, then there is the choice between taking a herbal laxative and using a small, warm water enema — about 1½ pints (850 ml) would be enough. This treatment will depend on whether there is someone to administer it — although it could be self-administered if the patient is confident about it.

Week Two, Day Three:
This is a progressive diet and the aim, throughout, is to increase the amount of raw foods taken, as these encourage healing and raise the level of health generally. When accompanied by whole cereals, vegetable and grain protein, unsaturated oils and natural sugars, a real balance is achieved. Individuals differ, of course, and in offering general advice, it is impossible to cater for special needs. The reader who feels the need of personal support should consult a qualified naturopath.

7 a.m. Herbal tea as before.
8 a.m. Fresh carrot juice.
8.30 a.m. Breakfast: 3 to 4 tablespoons of boiled rice

with 6 prunes or apricots, 2 tablespoons natural
yogurt and 1 tablespoon of ground almonds.

10.30 a.m. Barley Cup or similar.

12.30 p.m. Fresh carrot juice.

1 p.m. Lunch: 3 to 4 tablespoons of boiled brown rice
with 1 tablespoon of grated raw carrot, 1 teaspoon of
chopped parsley, 1 teaspoon of sunflower seeds, 6 to
8 sprigs of watercress, chopped and mixed into the
rice with 1 or 2 tablespoons of natural yogurt and a
small amount, say ½ teaspoon, of yeast extract.

3.30 p.m. China tea or herbal tea.

5.30 p.m. Carrot juice.

6.00 p.m. Evening meal: Brown rice, as before, mixed
with one grated raw apple including skin and pips,
soaked prunes or apricots, 1 tablespoon of ground
almonds and 2 tablespoons of natural yogurt (with a
little honey if necessary).

8.30 p.m. Barley Cup or peppermint tea.

9.30/10 p.m. Red grape juice as before.

Week Two, Day Four:
This is a repetition of Day Three. By now, considering
this is the second week, a definite lessening of
symptoms will be experienced and a little more energy
will be available. Certainly, the nervous system will be
calmer. Each day, the diet will get more interesting.

Week Two, Day Five:
The routine as before, with the waking drink and carrot
juice.

Breakfast: A grated raw apple, 4 to 6 prunes or apricots,
1 tablespoon of ground almonds, 2 tablespoons of
natural yogurt and a ripe banana.

Mid-morning: Barley Cup or dandelion coffee or apple
juice.

Before lunch: Tomato juice.

Lunch: 4 oz (115 g) cottage cheese, into which is mixed 1 teaspoon of chopped mint, 1 grated carrot, 1 teaspoon of sunflower seeds, 1 dessertspoon of raisins, 1 tomato (scalded and the skin removed), 1 teaspoon of cider vinegar and a few sprigs of watercress.

Mid-afternoon: Herbal or China tea or bottled fruit juice (apple or pineapple).

Before the evening meal: Carrot or tomato juice.

Evening meal: 2 potatoes (small), steamed with their skins on, 2 carrots (small), 2 oz (55 g) of frozen peas, 1 teaspoon of polyunsaturated margarine and 1 teaspoon of yeast extract.

Routine as before to finish the evening.

Week Two, Day Six:
Repeat Day Five.

Week Two, Day Seven:
Maintain the usual routine for between meals.

Breakfast: Muesli: Overnight, soak 2 tablespoons of flaked oats or wheat in 4 tablespoons of cold water. In the morning, add: 1 grated raw apple, 1 dessertspoon of raisins, 8 chopped almonds, 1 dessertspoon of powdered milk (or 2 tablespoons of yogurt) and 1 teaspoon of honey. Chew this really well.

Lunch: 2 or 3 lettuce leaves, 4 or 5 sprigs of watercress, 1 skinned tomato, 1 grated raw carrot, 1 small grated raw beetroot, sunflower seeds, ½ an apple, chopped or grated, 4 oz (115 g) cottage cheese, 2 teaspoons cider vinegar sprinkled over 1 or 2 steamed potatoes with skin still on.

Evening meal: Steamed vegetables: ¼ heart of cabbage (if not too big), 2 carrots, 1 small onion, ½ a red or green pepper, sliced into the cabbage and steamed together, 2 oz (55 g) grated Cheshire cheese to sprinkle over. (*Note:* Peppers are a rich source of vitamin C and retain quite an amount of it even when cooked.)

This completes the second week. Now make an assessment — weigh yourself. How successful have you been in your estimation? Are you pleased with your progress? Do you still feel hungry after meals? If so, this will pass as your stomach returns to normal size. As the meals become slightly more comprehensive, do you still suffer pain or flatulence? The flatulence may persist for weeks yet, but should be less severe in frequency and volume. Do you feel more relaxed and optimistic? Make a list of what yet needs to be achieved, and feel pleased and confident with your progress so far.

Week Three

Quite a number of changes will be made in the diet this week, progressing to a full normal reformed diet in the fourth week. These changes may be too rapid for some, and slight regression might occur. If this is the case, return to the stage that provided most comfort for a few more days and then try progression again. There is no merit in forcing on if it has a negative effect.

Week Three, Day One:
First thing: On waking, 2 teaspoons of cider vinegar and a little honey in hot water.
Before breakfast: 4 fl oz (120 ml) of bottled apple juice.
Breakfast: Muesli with prunes and yogurt.

11 a.m. Coffee-type drink.

Before lunch: Vegetable juice: choose from carrot, beetroot, celery, tomato, or a mixture of any two. Take 4 fl oz (120 ml) as usual.

Lunch: Salad: Keep amounts small. Use a sliced pepper, lettuce, watercress, beetroot, carrot, sunflower seeds, tomato, cottage cheese and mint. For the starch requirement have slice of 100 per cent wholewheat bread and polyunsaturated margarine. For dessert, an apple.

4 p.m. China or herb tea, as before.

Before the evening meal: Grapefruit juice.

Evening meal: Poached egg on mashed carrots with green vegetable in season, and a potato in its skin. For dessert, an apple or pear.

2 hours later: A coffee-type drink if needed.

Before bed: The usual grape juice.

Week Three, Day Two:

First thing: On waking, cider vinegar as before.

Before breakfast: Apple juice as before.

Breakfast: A banana, 8 almonds, 8 dates, an apple, yogurt or 4 fl oz (120 ml) untreated milk.

11 a.m. Grapefruit juice.

Before lunch: Mineral water.

Lunch: Salad mixture as before, but have 2 oz (55 g) milled nuts (not peanuts) as protein, and potato as starch. For dessert, an apple.

4 p.m. Tea as before.

Before the evening meal: Grapefruit juice.

Evening meal: Grilled white fish — haddock, cod or plaice fillet, with carrots and peas. For dessert, grapes or pear. Follow this with the usual bedtime drink.

Week Three, Day Three:
First thing: Early drinks as before.
Breakfast: A boiled egg, 1 slice of 100 per cent wholemeal bread with polyunsaturated margarine. One or two apples.
Mid-morning: Grapefruit juice.
Before lunch: Mineral water.
Lunch: Salad: Try different ingredients, e.g. celery or cucumber, 2 oz (55 g) Cheddar cheese, and 1 or 2 potatoes.
  For dessert, soaked prunes and/or apricots.
4 p.m. Tea as usual.
Before evening meal: Pineapple juice.
Evening meal: Millet and Tomato Savoury (page 69) with carrots, and green vegetables.
  For dessert, grapes or a pear.

To complete the week, repeat the three days already given, and then Day One again. If the diet has been adhered to and progress has been made the fourth week can be started with confidence.

Week Four
Monday:
First thing: Choose between cider vinegar, fruit juices and herb tea.
Before breakfast: Mineral water.
Breakfast: Natural yogurt with a little honey, an apple, 8 to 12 grapes and a pear. The yogurt can be eaten straight or the whole thing made into a fruit salad and the yogurt poured over.
Mid-morning: Savoury yeast extract drink diluted with milk and water; carrot juice or herb tea.
Before lunch: Pineapple juice.

Lunch: Salad: Lettuce, tomato (skinned), grated carrot and beetroot, a little sliced pepper, sprouted alfalfa seeds (see page 92), 2 small slices of 100 per cent wholewheat bread and unsalted butter. A hard-boiled egg. Use cider vinegar and sunflower oil as salad dressing or, alternatively, yogurt.

Fresh fruit as dessert.

Mid-afternoon: China tea.

Before the evening meal: Pineapple juice.

Evening meal: First course: Half an avocado with vinaigrette dressing.

Second course: Cauliflower, carrots, courgettes (in season), 2oz (55g) grated Cheddar cheese to sprinkle over the vegetables.

Fresh fruit to follow.

Evening drinks as before.

Tuesday:

Note: Before and between breakfast, lunch and the evening meal, drinks should follow the same pattern as before.

Breakfast: Soaked prunes and apricots, 1 teaspoon of sunflower seeds, 1 dessertspoon of ground almonds, natural yogurt.

Lunch: Salad: Watercress and orange, celery, beetroot. Dressing: Yogurt and Chopped Mint (page 82). Try potato and cottage cheese with this. Eat as much as you feel comfortable with.

Fresh fruit to follow.

Evening meal: First course: Avocado with vinaigrette dressing (page 82).

Second course: Mushroom omelette, peas or runner beans, and carrots.

Dessert: Apple Crumble (page 83).

Wednesday:
(Keep to the regular pattern of drinks.)

Breakfast: A boiled egg, 2 slices of 100 per cent wholemeal bread and polyunsaturated margarine, and an apple.

Lunch: Grated carrot, grated apple, grated raw beetroot 1 tablespoon of sunflower seeds, 1 teaspoon of chopped parsley, 4 oz (115g) of cottage cheese, 2 rye crispbreads and polyunsaturated margarine. French dressing. A *ripe* banana and yogurt to follow.

Evening meal: First course: Half a grapefruit. Second course: Cheesy Soya Mix (page 71), green vegetables (e.g. cabbage), carrots, leeks (in season) or onions. Dessert: Soaked prunes and apricots with goat's milk yogurt.

Thursday:
Breakfast: Home-made Muesli (page 65).
Lunch: Mixed salad: Lettuce, watercress, tomato (skinned), 1 small raw courgette — grated, grated carrot, a few raisins, a slice of onion, yogurt and mint dressing. A slice of 100 per cent wholewheat bread and butter, and 1 tablespoon of ground almonds.

Evening meal: First course: Tomato salad. Second course: Egg and Cheese Bake (page 70), with peas or runner beans, carrots and courgettes. Dessert: Fresh fruit.

Friday:
Breakfast: Fresh fruit: Grapes, an orange, an apple and a few dates and nuts, preferably almonds or hazelnuts.
Lunch: Salad: Sprouted alfalfa seeds, coleslaw or raw cabbage, carrots with a little onion, and vinaigrette dressing. One or two potatoes. Soaked prunes to follow.

Evening meal: First course: Half a grapefruit. Second course: Stuffed Pepper (page 77), carrots and green vegetables (in season). Dessert: Baked apples, stuffed with raisins or dates.

Saturday:

Breakfast: A sliced ripe banana, raisins, sunflower seeds and natural yogurt.

Lunch: Salad: Mixed cooked beetroot, diced and chopped celery, apple and walnuts tossed in vinaigrette dressing, two rye crispbreads with cottage cheese.

Fresh fruit — grapes or peaches (in season).

Evening meal: First course: Tomato salad.

Second course: Chestnut Pudding (page 75), with green vegetables, carrots and peas.

Dessert: Fresh fruit salad.

Sunday:

Breakfast: Scrambled eggs on toast and an apple.

Lunch: First course: Half a grapefruit.

Second course: Cauliflower cheese, courgettes and carrots.

Dessert: Baked apples.

Evening meal: Fresh fruit: An apple, an orange, grapes, nuts and raisins.

Weeks Five and Six

Menus for two weeks will help you to follow the previous regime, and give a framework to guide you for the future.

The drinks for taking first thing on waking will not be specially listed; to jog your memory, you may choose from:

Cider vinegar, hot water and honey,
Squeezed lemon juice, hot water and honey,
Herbal tea of choice — peppermint, chamomile, etc.,
Fruit juices — orange, apple, pineapple, etc.

The same thing applies to the bedtime drink. Choose from:
Slippery Elm Food,
Grape juice (red), hot or cold,
Vecon (with a dash of milk).

Note: Drinks should be ½ tumbler in quantity except first and last thing, when double the quantity is taken, and always *sipped*.

Monday:
Breakfast: Soaked prunes and natural yogurt.
Mid-morning: Vecon with dash of milk.
Lunch: Salad: grated carrot, watercress, ½ apple grated, tomato (scalded and skinned), sunflower seeds and raisins.
Dressing: Cider vinegar and sunflower oil. Baked jacket potato and a little butter, 2 tablespoons ground almonds.
Mid-afternoon: Herbal Tea, Rosehip, Peppermint or Chamomile.
Before evening meal: Pineapple juice.
Evening meal: Wholewheat macaroni, home-made tomato sauce (see page 78), steamed carrots and broccoli (or similar). Baked apple stuffed with dates.

Tuesday:
Breakfast: Grated raw apple with Muesli (page 65).
Mid-morning: Barley Cup (or similar).
Before lunch: Carrot juice.
Lunch: Salad: Lettuce, grated carrot, slice or two onion,

grated *raw* beetroot, mustard and cress, sunflower seeds.

Dressing: Yogurt and chopped parsley. 2 rye crispbreads and butter. Apple or pear to follow.

Mid-afternoon: Herbal tea.

Before evening meal: Pineapple juice.

Evening meal: Millet and Tomato Savoury (page 69), carrots and leeks. Soaked apricots and yogurt.

Wednesday:

Breakfast: Fresh fruit: grapes or pear.

Mid-morning: Vecon.

Before lunch: Pineapple juice.

Lunch: Salad: Lettuce, tomato (skinned), grated carrot and ½ apple, watercress, sunflower seeds and raisins; hard-boiled egg. Cider vinegar and oil dressing. Slice wholemeal bread and butter. Soaked apricots.

Mid-afternoon: Herbal tea.

Before evening meal: Carrot juice.

Evening meal: Vegetable and Lentil Casserole (page 72), cabbage. Apple Crumble (pages 83 and 84).

Thursday:

Breakfast: Soaked prunes and Muesli (page 65).

Mid-morning: Barley Cup.

Before lunch: Apple juice.

Lunch: Brown Rice Salad (page 81).

Mid-afternoon: Herbal tea.

Before evening meal: Carrot juice.

Evening meal: Omelette (tomato or mushroom), with peas (not tinned) and carrots. Baked apple with raisins.

Friday:
Breakfast: 2 slices wholemeal toast and butter, with honey.
Mid-morning: Vecon.
Before lunch: Apple juice.
Lunch: Brown Rice Salad (page 81).
Mid-afternoon: Herbal tea.
Before evening meal: Carrot juice.
Evening meal: Omelette (tomato or mushroom), with peas (not tinned) and carrots. Baked apple with raisins.

Saturday:
Breakfast: Soaked apricots and yogurt.
Mid-morning: Barley Cup.
Lunch: Salad: Lettuce, tomato (skinned), cucumber (unskinned), grated carrot, watercress, ½ orange segmented, sunflower seeds. Vinaigrette dressing (page 82). Baked jacket potato, a little butter. Fresh fruit.
Mid-afternoon: China tea: Lapsang or jasmine.
Before evening meal: Carrot juice.
Evening meal: Chestnut Pudding (page 75), with runner beans (in season) or greens of some sort and parsnips. Fruit Jelly (page 88).

Sunday:
Breakfast: Toast and butter and honey.
Mid-morning: Tomato juice with *Vecon.*
Before lunch: Apple juice.
Lunch: Cheesy Soya Mix (page 71), broad beans or greens, mashed swede. Baked jacket potato. Fresh fruit salad with natural yogurt and honey.
Mid-afternoon: China or herbal tea.
Before evening meal: Carrot juice.

Evening meal: Apple, pear, grapes; raisins (or dates), 12 almonds.

Monday:
Breakfast: Grated raw apple and muesli.
Mid-morning: Tomato juice with *Vecon*.
Before lunch: Apple juice.
Lunch: Salad: Coleslaw of carrot and apple, grated; chopped cabbage, chopped onion (to taste), sunflower seeds and raisins with dressing of yogurt, black pepper and cider vinegar, (chopped mint may be added in season). 2 rye crispbreads and butter. Apricot crumble.
Mid-afternoon: Tea. Herbal or China.
Before evening meal: Pineapple juice.
Evening meal: 1st course: Avocado with chopped mint and lemon juice.
    2nd course: Egg and Cheese Bake (page 70), carrots, runner beans or cabbage.
    Sweet: Baked apple or fresh fruit.

Tuesday:
Breakfast: Prunes or apricot and yogurt. Rye crispbread, butter and honey.
Mid-morning: Barley Cup.
Before lunch: Carrot juice.
Lunch: Salad: Lettuce, watercress, chopped celery and pepper (green or red) and apple, grated carrot, parsley, ground almonds (2 tablespoons). Baked jacket potato. Vinaigrette dressing (page 82). Bread and Butter Pudding (page 87).
Mid-afternoon: Tea as usual.
Before evening meal: Tomato juice.
Evening meal: Aduki Bean Hotpot (page 73), green vegetable. Pineapple (fresh or tinned in natural juice).

Wednesday:
Breakfast: Fruit: apple, orange, dates, almonds.
Mid-morning: Tomato juice with *Vecon* or *Barmene*.
Before lunch: Pineapple juice.
Lunch: Salad: Cottage cheese with chopped celery, grated carrot, chopped parsley, raisins — mixed together served with sprigs of watercress. Wholemeal bread and butter. Stewed apple.
Mid-afternoon: Tea.
Before evening meal: Carrot juice.
Evening meal: 1st course: Avocado Vinaigrette.
2nd course: Egg and Cheese Bake (page 70), with jacket potato and green vegetables (runner beans in season).
Sweet: Fruit jelly (page 88).

Thursday:
Breakfast: Branflakes and raisins. 1 apple.
Mid-morning: Barley Cup.
Before lunch: Pineapple juice.
Lunch: Salad: Lettuce, watercress, tomato, cucumber, grated carrot, sunflower seeds. Yogurt Mint Dressing (page 82). Grated Cheshire cheese (2 oz/55 g). Fresh fruit.
Mid-afternoon: Tea or fruit juice.
Before evening meal: Tomato or carrot juice.
Evening meal: Lentil Roast (page 74), leeks, green vegetables. Baked apple and raisins.

Friday:
Breakfast: ½ grapefruit, 1 pear, 8 dates, 8 almonds. Yogurt.
Mid-morning: Vecon and tomato juice.
Before lunch: Pineapple juice.
Lunch: Watercress and fresh orange segments with

yogurt and ground almonds. Rye crispbread. Bread and butter pudding.

Mid-afternoon: Tea or fruit juice.

Before evening meal: Carrot juice.

Evening meal: Stuffed peppers. Parsnips or carrots, green vegetables. Soaked apricots or prunes.

Saturday:

Breakfast: 2 slices wholemeal toast, butter and honey. 1 apple.

Mid-morning: Barley Cup.

Before Lunch: Pineapple juice.

Lunch: Rice salad with watercress. Rye crispbreads. Stewed apple.

Mid-afternoon: Tea (china or herbal).

Before evening meal: Carrot juice.

Evening meal: Savoury Jacket Potato (page 76), green vegetables. Fresh fruit salad and yogurt.

Sunday:

Breakfast: Branflakes and raisins. 1 apple.

Mid-morning: Barley Cup or *Vecon.*

Before lunch: Apple juice.

Lunch: Chestnut Pudding (page 75), carrots, green vegetables. Baked egg custard.

Mid-afternoon: The usual tea or fruit juice.

Before evening meal: Carrot juice.

Evening meal: Watercress sandwiches. Apple, pear, dates and nuts.

These menu plans should have given you an under-standing of how to continue dietetically. Apart from a possible increase in quantities, the overall pattern should remain similar. Care must be taken not to increase the quantities too much because of the risk that an over-full stomach may protrude through the oesophageal opening. By avoiding such pressure, and by eating wholesome nourishing foods, the chances of the hernia actually healing are greatly increased.

4.

EXERCISE

It was said in an earlier section that exercise not only keeps muscles in good tone, but affects the tissues throughout the body by rhythmical cell activity. Short bursts of exercise are really not helpful; and just to run through a few exercises for ten minutes daily only helps to keep the body flexible, (though this is good), without having any deeper effect on cell activity. It is this deeper effect that is necessary for treating hiatus hernia, as well as for improving the abdominal muscle tone.

A good walk is excellent for this purpose. It should last at least thirty to forty minutes, building up to an hour, if possible. At the beginning, it may be necessary for some individuals to be more cautious. It would be a mistake to take on a long walk if quite unprepared for it. A regular walk say for twenty minutes, is not without value, and the length can be gradually increased. This would be preferable to taking on the longer walk and getting overtired, and being put off from doing any more. If carried out in this way, walking produces a mild glow or sweat, which shows that the whole system is activated, and elimination is accelerated through the lungs and skin, leaving less toxic matter which clogs the body.

Getting rid of waste matter is always important to health, and it is because many people are unaware of this principle in its entirety, or are only taught to watch bowel action and thereby neglect the lungs and skin, that overloading so often occurs. Bowel action is frequently less than adequate as well, unfortunately. However, if a good diet and regular exercise are observed, all these inequalities rebalance themselves through the innate disposition of body cells, which are health-orientated.

Our bodies, then, are always working towards *health*. If we only learnt not to throw spanners in the works by bad diet and bad habits generally, the level of good health experienced would be much higher.

There are several specific exercises for the abdominal muscles, and these will be beneficial if practised regularly and rhythmically. It would probably be advisable to graduate the time factor for those who are weak or unfamiliar with exercising but, generally, fifteen to twenty minutes daily is the average time necessary for maximum effect. (The most important exercise — deep, diaphragmatic breathing — has already been described.)

The practice of these exercises, for ten minutes to begin with, increasing to twenty, will help specifically, but will also increase body awareness, and thereby improve posture. All too frequently, because of rushing, tiredness, and the effect of gravity, we tend to sink and slump down, nevertheless remaining tense at the same time. It is really important that we become aware of this and lift overselves up, as such exercise has both a physical and psychological effect, and is of great benefit. However, do not go to the other extreme and become rigid in the stretched up position! No, just lift the rib cage lightly, lowering and relaxing the shoulders, and stretching the back of the neck and top of the head easily. This immediately produces a feeling of greater control and integration and ability to cope with the daily round. So, the next time you feel 'down in the dumps', lift yourself up, remembering the slow deep breathing. The same type of exercise is effective if you feel jittery and 'up tight'.

It is surprising how much can be done, both to prevent illness and to promote good health. Health awareness presents an exciting challenge, and a basis for continual learning and personal development.

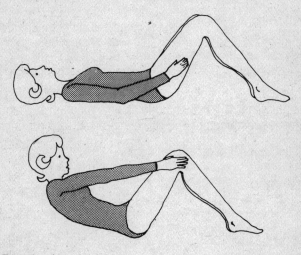

Exercise 1:
Lie in a crook position — that is, with both knees bent and feet close to buttocks and arms at the sides. Place hands on thighs where they join the abdomen, and then slide them up to reach the knees, lifting the head and shoulders, and breathing in slowly. Breathe out while falling back and relaxing. Repeat four to six times. Notice how the abdominal muscles shorten as you reach forward.

Exercise 2:
Lie flat on your back with legs out straight. Lift both legs together to 45°, breathing in slowly, then lower them, slowly breathing out and relaxing. Repeat four times.

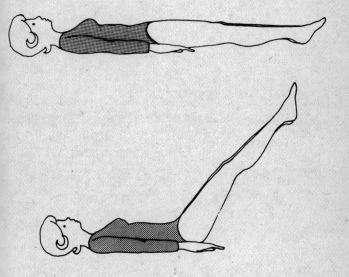

Exercise 3:
Sit on a stool, hands on hips. Use arms as levers, twisting round first to the right and then to the left. This movement takes place at the waist level. Look over each shoulder as you twist. Counting a right and left twist as one, repeat seven to ten times. No special breathing, but note that you do *not* have to hold your breath.

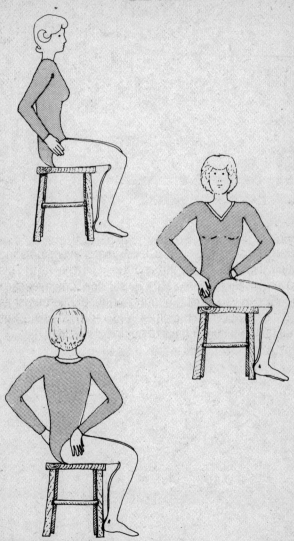

Exercise 4:
Sit on a straight-backed chair with back supported and bottom tucked well back — arms at the sides. Relax forward, *breathing out* (head to knees). Uncurl, inching your back up against the back of the chair until upright, *breathing in* slowly all the time. Remember to keep the head low until upright position is reached, and the back should be rounded and uncurling — not coming up in a stiff straight line. Repeat four times.

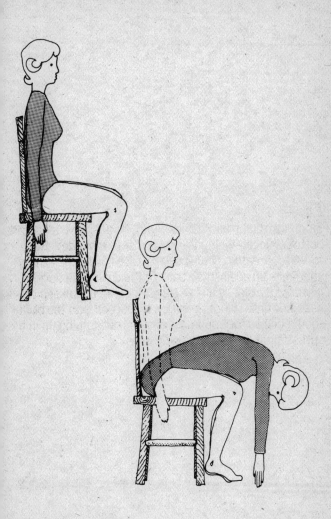

Exercise 5:
This one is designed to lift the rib cage and expand the
chest. Sit as in *Exercise 4.* Clasp hands behind the neck,
then drop head, shoulders and elbows forwards,
breathing out. Raise head and brace elbows back —
holding the chin in. Breathe in whilst raising up and
expanding. Repeat five times.

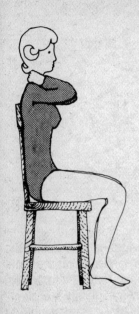

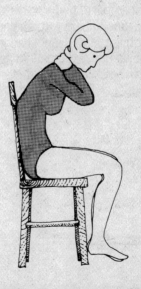

Exercise 6:
This one is designed for spine and chest mobility. Kneel in a 'donkey' position — on all fours, arms and thighs at right angles to body, spine straight. Bend head down; at the same time hump the spine (so that all is rounded) and breathe in. Now change by 'hollowing' the lower back and raising the head upwards. Breathe out as you do so. Keep elbows rigid as arms and thighs act as pillars of support. Repeat six times.

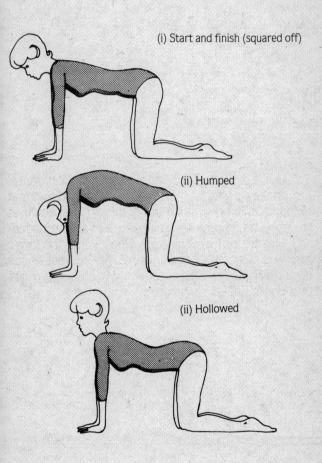

(i) Start and finish (squared off)

(ii) Humped

(ii) Hollowed

5.

OTHER NATURAL TREATMENTS

Hydrotherapy

Water is a source of natural healing which is usually undervalued. Cold water can have a tonic effect on blood vessels and nerves, especially in the skin. Hot water relaxes the body, but needs to be used with discretion. Hot and cold water, used in contrast, is very stimulating and beneficial in speeding up elimination, absorption and healing. Ice is useful in treating recent injuries, and prevents the body over-reacting to damage. Cold compresses to localized areas provide a natural warmth, which relaxes and promotes absorption and elimination of toxic matter. Thus, self-provided warmth is preferable to heat which is applied from outside the body. Water can be very useful in regulating body temperature by the application of complete body packs to promote sweating, or by repeated sponging to bring down a high temperature.

Water has been used as a therapy from ancient times — the Greeks and Romans both realized its value, externally and internally. They developed a form of colonic lavage, using an animal's horn to convey the water into the rectum. So enemas and colonic wash-outs are nothing new!

In addition, there are, or were, the spa towns, centres where people went to 'take the water' — to drink it, or bathe in it, or both. Unfortunately, most of the English centres have closed, but those on the continent seem to have been maintained.

The use of water in the case of hiatus hernia takes the form of cold packs applied to the upper abdominal area. The rationale behind this is that the pack promotes a temporarily increased circulation in the particular area of the diaphragm and stomach and thereby improves their action. Also, the absorption of cellular waste matter is accelerated, and muscle tone is improved.

The pack is applied for a minimum of three hours — but is ideally applied at bedtime and worn for the whole night. The immediate effect of the cold material on the skin and subcutaneous tissues is a contraction of the small blood vessels. This is followed very quickly by dilation, which is backed up by the deeper vessels, and general activity in the localized area is stimulated. After the first impact of cold, which should only last a few seconds, the pack should feel quite comfortable and gently warm. The frequency of application should be at least twice a week, regularly, for three weeks, at the beginning of the treatment.

To Make a Cold Pack:
You will need four to six layers of cotton or linen material (old sheeting or towelling) 7 inches (18 cm) square.
A piece of old woollen material or flannelette 9 inches (23 cm) square.
A large towel, folded lengthways to act as a binder.
3 large safety pins.

Method:

Soak the cotton material in cold water, wring out very well until only damp, and smooth out any creases. Apply to upper abdomen — that is, just where the ribs divide, above and including the umbilicus (navel). Cover with the larger piece of blanket, making sure good contact with the skin is made, and bind on with the folded towel, firmly but not too tightly. Pin in position; put on night wear and go to bed.

The pack should feel slightly warm — if not, two mistakes might have been made. (1) The pack may not have been wrung out sufficiently; (2) contact may be poor and air may be entering between the skin and pack. If neither of these is the case, then the vitality of the body is not yet strong enough to react properly and the pack should be discontinued, and tried later on in the treatment, say in two weeks' time. It is important that the pack becomes warm and does not stay cold and clammy — it is only being effective if it warms up within the first ten minutes of application. If this does not happen, it should be removed.

Note: No waterproofing material should be used, as this completely changes the effect of the pack, turning it into a poultice, which is not the effect wanted. When the pack is removed, after the three hours or in the morning as the case may be, the area should be washed with tepid water to remove traces of toxic matter, eliminated through the skin.

There are several other ways in which water can be used therapeutically; one is always to finish a hot bath or shower with a cold splash. Begin with the legs and feet, as being the less sensitive parts, and work up to the arms, abdomen and back. This can be done with a sponge, or with handfuls of water, or a shower attachment. Finish with a brisk rub down with a rough towel. Your whole body will be glowing and alive.

Some Extras For Temporary Use

Vitamin E: Wheatgerm oil capsules help in healing and in the better utilization of oxygen in the blood stream (100 IU strength, not more than three capsules daily). Discontinue after *six* weeks.

Herbal Tranquillizers: For the relief of tension, insomnia or general anxiety, a herbal tranquillizer, containing some of the B vitamins which help the nervous system, may be used.

Tissue Salts: The biochemical trace elements which help to activate and balance bodily reactions are also important in the treatment of hiatus hernia. Calcium fluoride, which enhances elasticity, is particularly valuable in this case. These salts are obtainable at health food stores and can be taken as directed. Neither the tissue salts nor the herbal tranquillizers should be taken for more than two months although, if necessary, either or both could be resumed after an interval. But the whole emphasis of natural treatment is to obviate the need for taking remedies, and to adjust the whole way of life to a healthy normality and balance.

6.

RECIPES

Breakfasts

HOME-MADE MUESLI
1 lb (455 g) oat, wheat or barley flakes
4 oz (115 g) raw cane sugar
4 oz (115 g) raisins
4 oz (115 g) chopped hazelnuts
2 oz (55 g) dried milk powder
8 dried apricots, chopped small
1 raw apple, grated

1. Mix dry ingredients together ready for use and store in an air-tight tin or jar.
2. Serve with grated raw apple. It is best to soak each portion in water overnight, adding the apple in the morning.

FRUIT AND NUT BREAKFAST
1 sweet apple
1 dessertspoon raisins
1 dessertspoon sunflower seeds
1 dessertspoon ground almonds

1. Thoroughly wash apple, grate on a coarse grater (skin and core as well), put into bowl and add other ingredients — mix up a little.
2. Eat slowly and chew well!

FRUITY YOGURT
4 oz (115 g) raisins or *sultanas*
1 large orange or *grapefruit*
¼ pint (140ml) natural yogurt

1. Wash raisins and drain — put into bowl and pour on boiling water to cover, stir and leave to soak overnight.
2. In the morning peel the orange and remove pith. Slice thinly with sharp knife.
3. Put into a dish and add the soaked raisins and yogurt.

Main Meals

CHESTNUT AND COURGETTE SAVOURY

Serves 2
3-4 medium courgettes
2 tablespoons sunflower oil
4 oz (115 g) tinned whole chestnuts
Pinch sea salt
1 teaspoon dried mixed herbs
2 eggs, beaten
1 teaspoon chopped fresh parsley

1. Wash and dry courgettes. Slice thinly.
2. Heat sunflower oil in a frying pan, tip in the sliced courgettes and toss about to brown them; add the drained chestnuts, stir about to warm them and add salt and dried herbs.
3. Pour over the beaten eggs, lower heat and allow to set. Sprinkle with parsley.
4. Serve with baked jacket potato and carrots.

NUTTY BEAN BAKE

Serves 3
4 oz (115 g) whole chestnuts
2 oz (55 g) coarsely ground hazelnuts
2 oz (55 g) pumpkin or sunflower seeds
2 oz (55 g) wholemeal breadcrumbs
½ teaspoon thyme
4 oz (115 g) aduki beans, soaked overnight
1 medium carrot, grated
2 eggs
Pinch sea salt

1. Combine the nuts, seeds, breadcrumbs and herb ingredients, drain aduki beans and add, also the grated carrot.
2. Add eggs one at a time and mix well with seasoning. Put into a greased baking dish.
3. Bake in a medium oven 375°F/190°C (Gas mark 5) for 35-45 minutes. Serve with green vegetables and Carrot Sauce (below).

Carrot Sauce
1. Liquidize 2 medium-sized carrots with juice of 1 lemon and pinch sea salt.
2. Put into pan and heat slightly — add 1 scant teaspoon agar powder *(Gelozone)* — bring to boil, stirring.
3. Pour over the savoury and serve.

SAVOURY APPLE PUDDING
Serves 3-4
4 oz (115 g) sunflower margarine
2 oz (55 g) ground almonds
4 oz (115 g) wholemeal breadcrumbs
4 oz (115 g) wholemeal plain flour
2 eggs, beaten
Sea salt and freshly ground black pepper
1 teaspoon dried sage
1 Bramley apple, coarsely grated
1 small onion, finely chopped

1. Soften and cream the margarine, fold in the ground almonds, crumbs and flour.
2. Add the eggs, seasoning, sage, apple and onion — combine well together.
3. Put into a greased basin, cover with greaseproof paper and a cloth tied down and steam for 1½ hours.
4. Serve hot with broccoli and carrots and apple sauce. Can be eaten cold with salad.

MILLET AND TOMATO SAVOURY
Serves 1
2 oz (55 g) millet
1 small tin (7 oz/200 g) tomatoes
1 clove garlic, crushed
2 teaspoons mixed herbs
½ level teaspoon yeast extract

1. Mix all ingredients together in a steel pan and simmer gently until the millet has absorbed all the moisture.
2. Stir fairly frequently.
3. Serve with green vegetables.

EGG AND CHEESE BAKE
Serves 2
2 eggs
¾ pint (425 ml) milk
1 teaspoon mixed herbs
2 oz (55 g) grated Cheddar cheese

1. Beat the eggs well. Add milk and stir in the other ingredients.
2. Put the mixture into a lightly oiled ovenproof dish and stand this in a larger pan with ½ inch (1 cm) of water.
3. Bake at 350°F/180°C (Gas Mark 4) for 45 minutes or until set.

CHEESY SOYA MIX

Serves 2
1 small onion, sliced
1 tablespoon sunflower seed oil
1 carrot, grated
2 oz (55 g) soya flakes
1 oz (30 g) ground almonds
2 oz (55 g) Cheddar cheese, grated
1 egg, beaten
1 teaspoon sage or mixed herbs
Water to mix, if necessary

1. Lightly fry the onion in the oil. Remove from heat.
2. Mix all the dry ingredients together in a bowl.
3. Stir in the onion, then the beaten egg.
4. If the mixture is still too dry to bind together, add a little water.
5. Cook in one of the following ways:
● Form into rissoles and fry in very little oil.
● Put the mixture into a lightly oiled ovenproof dish and bake at 375°F/190°C (Gas Mark 5) for 25-35 minutes.
● Put the mixture into a lightly oiled basin. Cover this with greaseproof paper and steam for 30-40 minutes.

VEGETABLE AND LENTIL CASSEROLE
Serves 2
1 onion or leek, chopped
1 tablespoon oil (sunflower, soya or olive)
2 large carrots, chopped small
2 sticks celery, chopped
2 small turnips or 1 small swede, chopped small
4 cabbage leaves, chopped
1 vegetable stock cube
1 teaspoon Vecon
½ pint (285 ml) boiling water
4 bay leaves
1 teaspoon mixed herbs
4 tablespoons lentils (green or brown)

1. Fry the onion (or leek) in the oil until lightly brown. Put into a casserole and add all the other vegetables.
2. Melt the stock cube and *Vecon* in the water, add herbs and bay leaves and pour over the vegetables.
3. Rinse the lentils in a sieve under the tap, and add to casserole. Mix in well. The ingredients should just be covered with liquid — if not, add a little more hot water.
4. Cover and cook in the oven at 350°F/180°C (Gas Mark 4) for 1½ hours.

ADUKI BEAN HOTPOT
Serves 2
1 onion
4 oz (115 g) aduki beans
2-3 carrots
1 tablespoon tomato purée
1 vegetable stock cube
1 pint (570 ml) boiling water
1 tablespoon oil
¼ teaspoon sea salt (optional)

1. Slice the onion and fry in the oil until browned. Place in a casserole dish.
2. Wash aduki beans, put into a pan, cover with water and bring to the boil. Boil for five minutes, then drain and discard the water.
3. Put the beans into the pot with the onion.
4. Chop the carrots small, then add to the pot.
5. Dissolve the stock cube in boiling water, add the tomato purée and pour over the other ingredients. Check the seasoning. If the stock cube was unsalted you may need to add a little salt.
6. Bake at 325°F/170°C (Gas Mark 3) for 1½ hours.

Variation:
Mung beans may be substituted for the aduki beans.

LENTIL ROAST

4 oz (115 g) brown or green lentils, cooked
1 oz (30 g) ground almonds
1 thick slice wholemeal bread, crumbled
1 onion, sliced
3 tablespoons oil
1 carrot
2 teaspoons mixed herbs
¼ teaspoon sea salt
Freshly ground black pepper
1 egg, beaten
Sesame seeds for garnish

1. Mix the lentils, almonds and breadcrumbs together.
2. Fry the sliced onion in 1 tablespoon of the oil until browned, and add to mixture.
3. Coarsely grate the carrot into the mixture, add the herbs and the rest of the oil. Mix well.
4. Add seasoning and beaten egg and mix again.
5. Put into a lightly oiled loaf tin. Press down and pattern the top with the back of a fork and bake at 375°F/190°C (Gas Mark 5) for 35 minutes, then at 400°F/200°C (Gas Mark 6) for 20 minutes.
6. Turn out onto a warmed plate and garnish with sesame seeds.

CHESTNUT PUDDING

1 tin (4 oz/115 g) chestnut purée
1½ oz (45 g) wholemeal breadcrumbs
1 small tin (7 oz/200 g) tomatoes
2 teaspoons mixed herbs
A little sea salt and freshly ground black pepper
2 tablespoons soya flour
1 small egg; beaten

1. Mix all the ingredients together (if too wet add a little more soya flour), and put the mixture into a greased basin.
2. Cover this securely with a cloth and steam it for 1 hour.
3. Turn the pudding out onto a dish and serve. This dish looks good surrounded by a ring of mashed carrots, and can be eaten hot with vegetables or cold with a salad.

Snacks and Light Meals

SAVOURY JACKET POTATO
(Ingredients per person)
½ onion
1 tomato, skinned
1 oz (30 g) grated Cheshire cheese
A little vegetable oil
1 hot baked potato

1. Slice onion and fry until translucent. Slice tomato and fry for 2 minutes with the onion.
3. Add cheese at the *last moment* so that it just melts a little.
4. Cut potato in half and pour on the filling, double it up again and serve with green vegetable.

TOMATOES AND ONIONS ON TOAST
1. Scald and skin 2 tomatoes and slice, peel and chop 1 small onion.
2. Put a knob of margarine in a pan and melt it. Add the chopped onion and brown lightly.
3. Add sliced tomatoes and ½ teaspoon mixed herbs. Cook 3-5 minutes.
4. Have ready 1 or 2 slices of toasted wholemeal bread — pile the tomato and onion mixture on and eat!

STUFFED PEPPERS
(Ingredients per person)
1 medium-sized pepper (red or green)
1 tablespoon brown rice
1 clove garlic, crushed
2 teaspoons of mixed herbs
1 carrot, grated
4 dried apricots, chopped

1. Cut off tops of peppers and remove the core and seeds — have an oven tin ready with ½ inch (2 cm) water to stand them in.
2. Wash and part-boil the rice in salted water for 15 to 20 minutes, then drain and mix in garlic, herbs, carrots and apricots.
3. Stuff this into the peppers and bake for 40-50 minutes at 375°F/190°C (Gas Mark 5) in the middle of the oven. Seasoning may be added sparingly.

AVOCADO AND CREAM CHEESE WITH MINT
Serves 2
1. Halve an avocado, sprinkle with cider vinegar; stuff with 2 oz (55 g) cream cheese.
2. Sprinkle with chopped mint (generously) and another shake of cider vinegar.
3. Eat with wholemeal bread and butter.

SPAGHETTI AND SIMPLE TOMATO SAUCE

Serves 2
4 oz (115 g) wholewheat spaghetti
7 oz (200 g) tin of tomatoes
1 garlic clove
1 teaspoon Barbados sugar
Pinch sea salt
1 teaspoon agar

1. Boil spaghetti in usual way in salted water, as directed on packet.
2. Prepare Tomato Sauce: Empty tin into small pan and chop tomatoes — add garlic and sugar, heat till nearly boiling then add agar. Cook 1 minute.
3. Serve with the spaghetti.

Salads

CHICORY, ORANGE AND AVOCADO 'SUNRISE'

1. Halve an avocado and remove flesh from the skin, chop into cubes.
2. Peel an orange, slice thickly and cut into cubes — mix with avocado, pile into centre of a small plate.
3. Arrange chicory leaves around (like sun rays) stuck into the mixture.
4. Sprinkle some chopped mint over if liked. Eat with wholemeal bread and butter.

PINEAPPLE, APPLE AND GINGER SALAD

2-3 apples
3 pieces stem ginger
12 oz (340 g) tin pineapple in its own juice
1 lettuce, washed
1 bunch watercress, washed
Vinaigrette (page 82)
1 tablespoon yogurt mixed with 1 tablespoon pineapple juice (more if necessary)
1 dessertspoon chopped mint
Flaked almonds

1. Dice apples finely. Chop ginger. Cut pineapple (if in rings) into chunks.
2. Tear up the lettuce, add sprigs of watercress and toss in french dressing. Spread out on a platter.
3. Mix pineapple, apple and ginger in the yogurt and pineapple juice. Pile onto lettuce and watercress base, sprinkle with mint and almonds.

BRUSSELS SPROUT, CELERY AND APPLE SALAD

1. Allow 4 large sprouts, 2 sticks of celery and ½ apple per person.
2. Prepare Sweet Salad Dressing (page 82).
3. On a board, with a sharp knife, chop sprouts and celery, coarsely or finely to taste.
4. Grate the apple coarsely, combine the salad ingredients, add dressing and decorate with either sultanas *or* sunflower seeds.

BEETROOT AND CELERY SALAD

1. Prepare Cottage Cheese Dressing (page 81).
2. Peel 2 cooked beetroots (globe type have the best flavour), slice and dice them, put into a large basin.
3. Take ½ head of celery, chop fairly small, omitting the tough outer sticks.
4. Mix with beetroot — add more celery if beetroot predominates.
5. Add the Cottage Cheese dressing — the mixture will go a pink colour.
6. Serve spoonfuls of salad on a bed of lettuce or watercress.

SPROUTED SALAD

Bean or alfalfa sprouts (see page 92)
Young dandelion leaves
Young nasturtium leaves
Mint or chives to flavour
Vinaigrette

1. Toss all the salad ingredients in vinaigrette. To make a colour contrast, grated carrot or sliced tomato can be added.

Salad Dressings:

COTTAGE CHEESE DRESSING
4 oz (115 g) cottage cheese
1 clove garlic, crushed
2-3 leaves fresh sage, chopped finely
3 tablespoons cider vinegar
1 tablespoon sunflower oil

1. Liquidize all together and refrigerate until needed.

BROWN RICE SALAD
(Serves 2)
4 oz (115 g) brown rice, washed
1 tablespoon vegetable oil
1 clove garlic, crushed
1 large carrot, grated
½ green pepper, finely chopped
1 teaspoon freshly chopped mint (or chives)
1 apple, diced
A few raisins
2 sticks celery, chopped
½ bunch watercress, cleaned and coarsely chopped
2 tablespoons coarsely ground or chopped nuts of choice
½ bunch watercress, cleaned, for garnish

1. Bring 1½ pints (850 ml) salted water to the boil, add the rice, oil and crushed garlic.
2. Simmer for 35 mins, stirring from time to time, then drain in a colander or sieve and allow to cool.
3. When the rice is cold — add other ingredients and mix well. Serve with rest of watercress as garnish.

VINAIGRETTE
2 tablespoons cider vinegar
1 tablespoon sunflower seed oil
1 clove of garlic, crushed
½ to 1 teaspoon honey
Any herb, to flavour

1. Mix all ingredients together.
2. Serve with any type of salad, or with avocado pears.

SWEET SALAD DRESSING
3 tablespoons cider vinegar
1 tablespoon sunflower oil
1 teaspoon honey
1 teaspoon mild mustard
1 tablespoon pineapple juice.

1. Liquidize all together — or put into a screw-top bottle or jar and shake vigorously.

YOGURT MINT DRESSING
1-2 teaspoons mint
¼ pint (140 ml) natural yogurt
1 level teaspoon honey

1. Mix all ingredients together.
2. Serve with salads.

Desserts

APPLE CRUMBLE I
(Serves 2)
2 cooking apples
1 dessertspoon raw cane sugar
1 lemon, grated rind and juice
4 oz (115 g) 100 per cent wholemeal flour
1 tablespoon raw cane sugar
2 oz (55 g) polyunsaturated margarine

1. Core the apples and grate them, together with skin, into an ovenproof dish.
2. Add the juice and grated rind of the lemon, and the sugar. Mix gently.
3. Top this mixture with the flour, sugar and margarine, mixed and rubbed together to form fine breadcrumbs.
4. Press down slightly over the apple mixture.
5. Bake at 400°F/200°C (Gas Mark 6) for 20-30 minutes.

APPLE CRUMBLE II
(Serves 2)

Apple Mix:
2-3 large cooking apples
Pinch cloves, cinnamon or grated lemon rind to flavour
1-2 tablespoons dark raw cane sugar

1. Peel and slice the apples. Arrange in a baking dish.
2. Sprinkle with the flavouring of your choice, to taste, plus the sugar.

Topping:

3 heaped tablespoons 100 per cent wholemeal flour
1 level tablespoon raw cane sugar
1 level tablespoon ground almonds
3 oz (85 g) unsalted butter

1. Mix the dry ingredients together, and chop in the butter. Rub in to a fine breadcrumb consistency.
2. Sprinkle over the apples to form a crust and press down lightly. Bake at 400°F/200°C (Gas Mark 6) for 30-40 minutes.

SULTANA SCONES

4 oz (115 g) sunflower margarine
8 oz (225 g) wholemeal plain flour
2 oz (55 g) soft raw cane sugar
2 oz (55 g) sultanas
Milk and yogurt to mix

1. Rub the fat into the flour until the mixture resembles breadcrumbs, cut in the sugar and sultanas;
2. Using 1 tablespoon milk with 1 dessertspoon natural yogurt mixed together, moisten the dry mixture, stirring with a knife. If necessary, use more liquid to reach a state where the dough can be kneaded into a ball.
3. Put onto floured board and, with knuckles, gently press out to ½-¾ inch (1.5-2 cm) thickness. Remember that, as no raising agent is used, these scones will remain the same height as when put into oven.
4. Cut out with a pastry cutter and bake in hot oven 400°F/200°C (Gas Mark 6) for 25 mins.

FLAPJACKS

6 oz (170 g) sunflower margarine
4 oz (115 g) black treacle
2 oz (55 g) Demerara sugar
8 oz (225 g) rolled oats
2 oz (55 g) walnuts or hazelnuts
4 oz (115 g) sultanas

1. Melt fat, treacle and sugar gently in a pan, then stir in other ingredients and blend well.
2. Turn onto a greased baking tin, press down evenly and bake at 375°F/190°C (Gas Mark 5) for 30-35 mins.
3. Mark into squares or fingers while still hot. Cool on wire tray. When cold, break into pieces.

STEAMED SULTANA PUDDING

(Serves 2)
2 oz (55 g) unsalted butter
2 oz (55 g) dark raw cane sugar
1 large egg, beaten
4 oz (115 g) 100 per cent wholemeal plain flour
Grated rind of 1 lemon
2 oz (55 g) sultanas, well washed

1. Lightly oil a pudding basin.
2. Cream the butter and sugar together, beat in the egg, then fold in the flour and lemon rind, then sultanas. Mix should be of dropping consistency: if too stiff, add a little lemon juice and water.
3. Put into the basin, cover with greaseproof paper and a cloth and tie these on firmly or use lid if the basin has one. Put into pan with 2 inches (50 cm) boiling water coming half-way up sides of basin. Boil *gently* for 1 hour — topping up with more boiling water at times and keep it to the half-way mark.
4. Serve with a sprinkling of sesame or sunflower seeds.

BREAD AND BUTTER PUDDING
(Serves 2)
2 large slices wholemeal bread, buttered
2 oz (55 g) sultanas or raisins, well washed
1 egg, beaten
½ pint (285 ml) milk
1 tablespoon raw cane sugar

1. Lightly butter an ovenproof dish. Cut up bread and butter to line the bottom and sides of the dish. Sprinkle with sultanas or raisins.
2. Beat the egg, milk and sugar together and pour over.
3. Bake in the oven at 350°F/180°C (Gas Mark 4) for 40 minutes, then raise heat to 400°F/200°C (Gas Mark 6) for 10 minutes, to brown the top of the pudding.

FRUIT JELLY

This can be made with fresh or dried fruits. Apples, pears, oranges, bananas — singly or mixed; or prunes, apricots, raisins — previously soaked of course.

1. Prepare the fruit in individual bowls or dish — either coarsely grate or chop the apple or pear; thickly slice the banana; segment and cut up the orange.
2. For each ½ pint (285 ml) fluid (water or juice) you will need a level teaspoon of agar-agar or *Gelozone*. The liquid must be boiled, but allow it to cool before pouring over the fruit.
3. The powder for the jelly can either be mixed to a paste with cold water and the rest added gradually, or sprinkled onto the water as it warms up — *not* when it has boiled.
4. Sugar or honey can be added to taste.

Note: These jellies don't turn out very well — so individual dishes or a large bowl are best.

ALMOND CAKE

4 oz (115 g) sunflower margarine (or similar)
2 tablespoons sunflower oil
4 oz (115 g) soft raw cane sugar
3 eggs
6 oz (170 g) wholemeal plain flour
2 oz (55 g) soya flour
2 oz (55 g) ground almonds
2-5 drops natural almond essence (optional)
2 oz (55 g) flaked almonds

1. Prepare a 7 inch (18 cm) cake tin.
2. In a large bowl, or mixer, cream the fat, oil and sugar.
3. Add eggs one by one, using a little of the flours (which have been sifted together along with the ground almonds) to prevent curdling.
4. Fold in remaining flour mix — add the essence (if used) and half the flaked almonds.
5. Put into the prepared tin, leaving the centre slightly hollowed to allow for rising; sprinkle over the rest of the flaked almonds.
6. Bake in centre of oven at 375°F/190°C (Gas Mark 5) for 1¼ hours. Cover with greaseproof paper but remove this for final ½ hour.

Variation: This mixture can be used to make small buns, using patty tins.

OLD-FASHIONED RICH FRUIT CAKE

4 oz (115 g) unsalted butter
2 oz (55 g) sunflower margarine
2 tablespoons sunflower oil
2 oz (55 g) soft raw cane sugar
1 tablespoon light-flavoured honey
8 oz (225 g) wholemeal plain flour
2 oz (55 g) soya flour
2 oz (55 g) ground almonds
4 eggs
Rind and juice of 1 large lemon
4 oz (115 g) sultanas
2 oz (55 g) currants
4 oz (115 g) raisins
2 oz (55 g) chopped apricots
Flaked almonds to decorate

1. Prepare a 7 inch (18 cm) cake tin.
2. Cream the butter, margarine, oil, sugar and honey.
3. Sift flours and almonds together, but do not add to the creamed mixture yet.
4. Beat eggs, gradually add the beaten eggs to the creamed mix, using a little flour to prevent curdling. Continue until all the eggs have been added.
5. Now fold in the remaining flour, grate in the lemon rind and add the juice, add the fruits mixing well with a lifting (folding) movement. The consistency of the mix should be 'soft dropping', i.e., it drops from the spoon easily, without being too wet.
6. Transfer mixture to baking tin. Sprinkle flaked almonds over the top.
7. Cover with greaseproof paper and bake in medium oven 350°F/180°C (Gas Mark 4) for 1 hour, then remove cover, raise temperature to 375°F/190°C (Gas Mark 5) for 30-40 mins.

Note: A change of flavour can be made by using black treacle instead of honey, and substituting 2 teaspoons of mixed spice instead of the lemon *rind* (the juice will still be needed).

LUNCH CAKE
1 cup All Bran
1 cup mixed fruit
1 cup soft brown sugar
1 cup milk
1 cup wholemeal flour

1. Soak the *All Bran*, mixed fruit and sugar overnight in the milk.
2. Next day, stir in the flour.
3. Bake in a loaf tin at 350°F/180°C (Gas Mark 4) for 45 minutes.

Note: Very tasty spread with margarine or butter.

Miscellaneous:

Making Juices Without a Juicer

This method could be used for root vegetables or any fruit that can be grated. You will need a soup plate or shallow dish, and a piece of gauze or muslin about 12 inches (35 cm) square, and a grater.

1. Arrange the muslin in the dish, grate the vegetable or fruit into it, then gather up the muslin carefully and squeeze out the juice from the pulp.
2. Transfer the juice to a cup or mug and dilute it with one tablespoonful of water. Drink (sip) at once. (4 fl oz/100 ml is the required amount.)

Note: Carrot, beetroot and apple can be frequently used, and perhaps less frequently, because of their unusual taste, potato, swede and turnip.

Sprouting Seeds, Grains and Beans

1. Use a clear jar covered with gauze and secured by a rubber band.
2. Put about 1 dessertspoonful of whatever seeds or grains you choose into the jar, and rinse well with cold water — no residue should be left in the jar.
3. Put on the gauze lid. Each day, rinse the seeds (it can be done through the lid without removing it) and drain well.
4. Sprouts appear after three to six days. Allow them to grow to 1 or 1½ inches (2.5-4 cm), then remove from the jar and eat both the seeds and the sprouts.
5. Begin the process again.

Some examples to try are:

Beans	*Seeds*	*Grains*
Aduki	Alfalfa	Wheat
Mung	Mustard	Rye
Chickpeas	Cress	Barley
Soya	Fennel	
Haricot	Sesame	
Black-eyed	Beet	
	Carrot	

Notes on Food Combinations

Some vegetables are notorious for causing disturbances in the digestive tract, and of course, this varies from person to person; but the generally accepted offenders are:

Cauliflower
Brussel Sprouts
Onions
Parsnips
Turnips
Cucumber

The first two vegetables should *always* be under-cooked, this prevents the over-production of sulphur in them, which is the cause of the trouble in the body. When any of these vegetables are eaten, it is better not to serve potatoes at the same meal.

Potatoes and all meat protein should be separated. If meat is eaten, carrots and green vegetables are the best combination. Jacket potatoes can be eaten with salads and with vegetarian dishes — but not with pasta, as this would be too starch-concentrated.

The combination of fresh fruit and starch should be avoided, this causes fermentation, and gas formation nullifies the vitamin content of the fruit, and slows digestion and absorption. Dried fruits and bananas, however, can be combined with starch.

The salad vegetables most complained about are cucumber, watercress and radishes. Eaten in small quantities in a mixed salad (using *one* of the above at a time) and without drinking at the same time, these can be digested comfortably — given that they are well-chewed. So there should be no problems if the advice on chewing (see page 24) is followed, and some of the recipes used.

It should be noted that baking powder is not used in any recipe. I never use baking powder and similar raising agents, because they inhibit the absorption of vitamins B, and are irritant to the gut. Therefore, recipes containing baking powder are avoided — or an extra egg is substituted where suitable. This is a good reason for avoiding shop cakes and biscuits as they usually contain baking powder, as well as other chemicals to colour and flavour.

INDEX